The Nuremberg Code

75th Anniversary Commemorative Edition

Commentary by
Vera Sharav

Introductory notes by
Ken McCarthy

B
Brasscheck
Press

KenMcCarthy.com

Copyright © 2022 Kenneth J. McCarthy

"Unless All Of Us Resist, Never Again Is Now"
Copyright © 2022 Vera Sharav.
Used by permission of Vera Sharav.

All rights reserved. No portion of this book may be reproduced in any form without permission from the publisher, except as permitted by U.S. copyright law.
For permissions contact: Books@Brasscheck.com

Medical Disclaimer
It is not the intention of any of the authors of this publication to offer medical advice. If you believe you need the services of a licensed health care practitioner, please seek one out.

Printed in the United States of America.

2nd Edition

Brasscheck Press
P.O. Box 145
Tivoli, NY
Brasscheck.com

The Nuremberg Code

75th Anniversary Commemorative Edition

Commentary by

Vera Sharav

Introductory notes by
Ken McCarthy

Publisher's Note

I'm writing this in early August of 2022.

My colleague Vera Sharav recently informed me that this month is the 75th anniversary of the publication of the Nuremberg Code.

I went to Google and typed in the search phrase "Nuremberg Code 75th Anniversary" and up came...nothing.

By way of comparison, I searched another anniversary this year, the 70th anniversary of the role Elizabeth Alexandra Mary Windsor is playing as Queen Elizabeth, and up came, in Google's words, "about 26,500,000 results."

I'm puzzled.

If you're someone interested enough in the Code to have acquired this book, I imagine you are too.

Some may consider the Nuremberg Code to be a technical document of interest to specialists only - I'll address that in a moment - but if that's the case, where are the specialists?

There is a field called "medical ethics." People in this field are called "medical ethicists" and they are employed by colleges, universities, government offices, health agencies, private practices, and health care facilities. They also work for pharmaceutical companies.

According to Salary.com, as of December 2021 clinical ethicists make a median salary of $102,977 and those working as professors of medical ethics earn a median salary of $150,983.

As of 2022, there are thirty-six colleges in the U.S. that offer degrees in Bioethics/Medical Ethics.

By one system of ranking, these are the top ten: 1) Harvard University, 2) Duke University, 3) Columbia University, 4) University of Pennsylvania, 5) Northwestern University, 6) Wake Forest University, 7) University of Richmond, 8) Creighton University, 9) Johns Hopkins University, and 10) Albany Medical College.

In the United States, the profession has its own association, the American Society for Bioethics and Humanities (ASBH) with nearly 1,800 members.

A search of the association's website yielded no results for "Nuremberg Code 75th Anniversary." However, five years ago in 2017, which I think all will agree was a different political climate, "Nuremberg Code 70th Anniversary" did yield a result. It was the topic of the keynote for the ASBH's annual convention.

I searched the websites of the ten universities listed above, who are the academic leaders of the study of medical ethics, and Google returned zero results. Two years ago, many of these same universities did note the 75th anniversary of the start of the Nuremberg Trials, so they are aware of the calendar and are capable of organizing events to mark important anniversaries.

I then reached out to the public relations departments of the FDA (15,100 employees), CDC (10,899 employees), and NIH (20,262 employees) to see if they have any events or press announcements on the anniversary scheduled. The CDC maintains a 200,000 square foot Global Communications and Training Center in Atlanta, where they employ dozens of full time employees to churn out press releases and audio visual programs - so I made a special point to contact them. I also reached out to Christine Grady's office. Grady is Head of the Department of Bioethics at NIH and the wife of Dr. Anthony Fauci. I thought that given NIH's substantial annual investment in public relations, and her family's obvious commitment to public dialogue, the NIH might be doing something.

It turns out that no one I communicated with at any of these institutions could point me to a single document or event that recognizes the significance of this year.

I do note that on April 28, 2022 New York College of Medicine and Touro University did co-sponsor a symposium on the 75th Anniversary of the Nuremberg Doctors' Trial which included some discussion of the Code which emanated from it, but this is literally the only event, talk, paper, article, news item, or panel discussion I could find anywhere on the Internet where this anniversary is mentioned, and even here it was mentioned only indirectly as a side issue.

You would think that one of the academic programs that trains medical ethicists or one of the large federal bureaucracies that employs them (FDA, CDC, NIH) might have found the time to dedicate some of its bandwidth to drawing attention to the Code and its importance, but as my research shows this has not been the case.

In fairness, they've probably been busy wrestling with pressing contemporary medical ethics issues - like employers requiring employees, who have natural immunity to a disease, to expose themselves to the risk of receiving repeated vaccinations against that disease as a condition of their continued employment. You can search the websites of the medical ethics programs at these institutions to see the level of resources they've applied to issues like this.

Based on the evidence above, I believe it's fair to say that for whatever reason the professional medical ethics community does not find the 75th anniversary of the Nuremberg Code terribly interesting.

If the professionals who draw salaries and consume tax dollars in pursuit of medical ethics are not interested, then why should we be?

A fair question - and the answer is in the Code itself.

Drafted at the conclusion of a series of trials of Nazi doctors who'd been charged of crimes - like murder and falsifying death certificates on behalf of their employer, the German government - the Nuremberg Code was the 20th century's most important and most high profile attempt to articulate specific ethical guidelines to protect patients from systematic abuse by doctors, health care practitioners, and medical systems.

The Code was drafted in response to the horror of an entire country's medical system being politicized, and "science" being used to justify mass crimes against humanity in which physicians played a key role. After the Nazi government's imposition of the Nuremberg Race Laws in 1935, Jewish doctors and medical professors were removed from their posts and replaced with card-carrying Nazi party members. In fact, according to Robert Jay Lifton's book "The Nazi Doctors," no profession had a higher percentage of Nazi party members than the medical profession.

Until the publication of the book you now hold in your hand, it was impossible to buy a book or download an eBook that was produced specifically for the purpose of making sure every human being has the opportunity to hold this important document in their own hands.

We are currently working on a second book with the provisional title: "The Nuremberg Code and Its Modern Enemies" where we will explore potential reasons why the 75th anniversary of the Code was almost universally ignored by the medical ethics profession, and why, starting in 2020, attempts to undermine the Code's authority have become a cottage industry for literally dozens of writers.

- Ken McCarthy
August 4, 2022

TABLE OF CONTENTS

Publisher's Note - Ken McCarthy .... *i*

"Unless All Of Us Resist, Never Again Is Now"
-Vera Sharav *1*

The Nuremberg Code *11*

Translations:

Hebrew *31*

German *33*

Chinese *37*

Hindi *39*

Spanish *41*

French *43*

Arabic *45*

Russian *47*

Portuguese *49*

Italian *51*

Japanese *53*

Additional Reading... *55*

Next Steps *57*

"Unless All Of Us Resist, Never Again Is Now"
-Vera Sharav

Full Speech - Nuremberg, August 20, 2022

"I came to Nuremberg to provide historical context to the current global threat confronting our civilization. These past two and a half years have been especially stressful – as painful memories were rekindled.

In 1941, I was three and a half when my family was forced from our home in Romania and deported to Ukraine.

We were herded into a concentration camp – essentially left to starve. Death was ever-present. My father died of typhus when I was five.

In 1944, as the Final Solution was being aggressively implemented, Romania retreated from its alliance with Nazi Germany. The government permitted several hundred Jewish orphans under the age of 12 to return to Romania. I was not an orphan; my mother lied to save my life.

I boarded a cattle car train – the same train that continued to transport Jews to the death camps – even as Germany was losing the war.

Four years elapsed before I was reunited with my mother.

The Holocaust serves as the archetypal symbol of unmitigated evil:
– Moral norms and human values were systematically obliterated.
– The Nazi system destroyed the social conscience.
– Millions of people were worked to death as slave laborers.
– Others were abused as experimental human guinea pigs.

The Holocaust did not begin in the gas chambers of Auschwitz and Treblinka.

The Holocaust was preceded by 9 years of incremental restrictions on personal freedom, and the suspension of legal rights and civil rights.

The stage was set by fear-mongering and hate-mongering propaganda.

A series of humiliating discriminatory government edicts demonized Jews as "spreaders of disease." We were compared to lice.

The real viral disease that infected Nazi Germany is Eugenics:
- Eugenics is the elitist ideology at the root of all genocides.
- Eugenics is cloaked in a mantle of pseudo-science.
- It was embraced by the academic and medical establishment as well as the judiciary – in Germany and the United States.

Eugenicists justify social and economic inequality.

They legitimize discrimination, apartheid, sterilization, euthanasia, and genocide. The Nazis called it "ethnic cleansing" for the protection of the gene pool.

Medicine was perverted from its healing mission and was weaponized.

First, it was to control reproduction through forced sterilization; then it was to eliminate those deemed to be "sub-human" – Untermenschen.

The first victims of medical murder were 1,000 disabled German infants and toddlers. This murderous operation was expanded to an estimated 10,000 children up to age 17.

The next victims were the mentally ill; they were followed by the elderly in nursing homes. All of these human beings were condemned as "worthless eaters."

Under Operation T-4, designated hospitals became killing stations where various extermination methods were tested – including Zyklon B, the gas that was used in the death camps.

The objective of the Nazi Final Solution was to annihilate the entire 11 million people of the Jewish Population of Europe as quickly and efficiently as possible.

The Nazis enacted discriminatory laws; they utilized modern technology; low-cost industrial methods; an efficient transportation system; and a highly trained bureaucracy that coordinated the industrial genocidal process. The objective was high speed, maximum efficiency at the lowest cost.

The human casualties of this unprecedented genocide were 6 million Jews and 9 million other people whom the Nazis dehumanized as Untermenschen.

The purpose of Holocaust memorials is to warn and inform future generations about how an enlightened, civilized society can be transformed into a genocidal universe ruled by absolute moral depravity.

If we are to avert another Holocaust, we must identify ominous current parallels before they poison the fabric of society.

Since the Nazi era, the study of history and most of the humanities – including philosophy, religion, and ethics – has been overshadowed by an emphasis on utilitarian science and technology.

As a result, few people recognize the foreboding similarities between current policies and those under the Nazi regime.

By declaring a state of emergency, in 1933 and in 2020, constitutionally protected personal freedom, legal rights, and civil rights were swept aside. Repressive, discriminatory decrees followed.

In 1933, the primary target for discrimination were Jews. Today, the target is people who refuse to be injected with experimental, genetically engineered vaccines. Then and now, government dictates were crafted to eliminate segments of the population.

In 2020, government dictates forbade hospitals from treating the elderly in nursing homes. The result was mass murder.

Government decrees continue to forbid doctors to prescribe life-saving, FDA-approved medicines; government-dictated protocols continue to kill.

The media is silent – as it was then.

The media broadcasts a single, government-dictated narrative – just as it had under the Nazis. Strict censorship silences opposing views.

In Nazi Germany few individuals objected; those who did were imprisoned in concentration camps.

Today, doctors and scientists who challenge the approved narrative are maligned; their reputations trashed. They risk losing their licenses to practice, as well as having their homes and workplaces raided by SWAT teams.

The moral significance of the Nuremberg Code cannot be overstated:

The Nuremberg Code is the most authoritative, internationally recognized document in the history of medical ethics.

This landmark document was formulated in response to the evidence of medical atrocities committed by Nazi physicians and scientists.

The Code sets forth moral boundaries for research involving human beings.

The Nuremberg Code rejects the ideology of Eugenics and unequivocally asserts the primacy and dignity of the individual human being – as opposed to "the greater good of society."

American jurists who formulated the Nuremberg Code incorporated the official 1931 German "Guidelines for Human Experimentation" authored by Dr. Julius Moses. Those Guidelines remained legally in force until 1945. The Nazis violated them in their entirety. Dr. Moses, who was Jewish, was deported to Theresienstadt where he died.

The Nuremberg Code defined foundational, universal moral and legal standards, affirming fundamental human rights.

These human rights apply to every human being.

The Code sets limits on the parameters of permissible medical experiments.

Equally important, the Nuremberg Code holds doctors and research investigators personally responsible to ensure the human subjects' safety, and to ensure that the person freely gives his voluntary, fully-informed consent. The standards of the Nuremberg Code are incorporated in the International Criminal Code. They are legally applicable today – in peacetime and during war.

The objective of the Nuremberg Code is to ensure that medicine never again deviates from the precautionary ethical principle: "First, do no harm."

The Nuremberg Code has served as a blueprint for subsequent national and international codes of human rights – to ensure that the rights and dignity of human beings are upheld; and to ensure that medical doctors never again engage in morally abhorrent experiments.

Like the 10 Commandments, not a word of the Code may ever be changed.

The first of the 10 ethical principles lays down the foremost ethical requirement – which is spelled out in great detail:

"The voluntary consent of the human subject is absolutely essential".

"This means that the person involved should have legal capacity to give consent; should be so situated as to be able to exercise free power of choice, without the intervention of any element of force, constraint, or coercion; and should have sufficient knowledge and comprehension of the elements of the subject matter involved as to enable him to make an understanding and enlightened decision. This requires that before the acceptance of an affirmative decision by the experimental subject [he] should be [informed of] the nature, duration, and purpose of the experiment; the method and means by which it is to be conducted; all inconveniences and hazards reasonably to be expected; and the effects upon his health or person which may possibly come from his participation in the experiment.

The duty and responsibility for ascertaining the quality of the consent rests upon each individual who initiates, directs, or engages in the experiment. It is a personal duty and responsibility which may not be delegated to another with impunity."

The genocidal culture that permeated the Nazi regime did not end in 1945. It metastasized in the United States.

At the end of the war, US government agents helped 1,600 high-ranking Nazi scientists, doctors, and engineers to evade justice at Nuremberg.

These Nazi technocrats facilitated the murderous Nazi operations. They were Hitler's partners in crimes against humanity. They were secretly smuggled into the US under Operation Paperclip. This was in violation of explicit orders by President Harry Truman. These Nazi criminals were placed in high-level positions at major American scientific and medical institutions where they continued their work.

What's more, these Nazi technocrats trained a generation of American scientists, doctors, and engineers. This is how Nazi methods, and the immoral disregard for human values were entrenched in America.

In 1961, in his farewell address to the nation, President Dwight Eisenhower warned against the increasing dominance of "the military-industrial complex" whose "total influence – economic, political, even spiritual – is felt [everywhere]." Eisenhower warned: "we must be alert to the danger that public policy could itself become the captive of a scientific-technological elite."

In May 2022, at the World Economic Forum in Davos, Klaus Schwab, the architect of the dystopian Great Reset, declared: "Let's be clear, the future is not just happening; the future is built by us, a powerful community here in this room. We have the means to impose the state of the world."

The ultimate goal of these megalomaniacs is to gain total control of the world's natural resources, financial resources, and to replace humans with Transhuman robots.

Transhumanism is a bio-tech-enhanced caste system – the New Eugenics.

Klaus Schwab's lead advisor is Yuval Noah Harari, an Oxford University trained, Israeli. Harari is a proponent of the New Eugenics and Transhumanism.

Harari refers to humans as "hackable animals." He declared: "We have the technology to hack humans on a massive scale…"

Harari despises the very concept of God.

Transhumanists despise human values, and deny the existence of a human soul. Harari declares that there are too many "useless people." The Nazi term was "worthless eaters."

This is the New Eugenics.

It is embraced by the most powerful global billionaire technocrats who gather at Davos: Big Tech, Big Pharma, the financial oligarchs, academics, government leaders and the military industrial complex. These megalomaniacs have paved the road to another Holocaust.

This time, the threat of genocide is Global in scale.

This time instead of Zyklon B gas, the weapons of mass destruction are genetically engineered injectable bioweapons masquerading as vaccines.

This time, there will be no rescuers.

Unless All of Us Resist, Never Again is Now."

Vera Sharav
Holocaust Survivor
Public Advocate for Human Rights
Founder and President of the Alliance for Human Research Protection
www.AHRP.org

The Nuremberg Code

1.

The voluntary consent of the human subject is absolutely essential.

This means that the person involved should have legal capacity to give consent; should be so situated as to be able to exercise free power of choice, without the intervention of any element of force, fraud, deceit, duress, overreaching, or other ulterior form of constraint or coercion; and should have sufficient knowledge and comprehension of the elements of the subject matter involved, as to enable him to make an understanding and enlightened decision.

This latter element requires that, before the acceptance of an affirmative decision by the experimental subject, there should be made known to him the nature, duration, and purpose of the experiment; the method and means by which it is to be conducted; all inconveniences and hazards reasonably to be expected; and the effects upon his health or person, which may possibly come from his participation in the experiment.

The duty and responsibility for ascertaining the quality of the consent rests upon each individual who initiates, directs or engages in the experiment. It is a personal duty and responsibility which may not be delegated to another with impunity.

2.

The experiment should be such as to yield fruitful results for the good of society, unprocurable by other methods or means of study, and not random and unnecessary in nature.

3.

The experiment should be so designed and based on the results of animal experimentation and a knowledge of the natural history of the disease or other problem under study, that the anticipated results will justify the performance of the experiment.

4.

The experiment should be so conducted as to avoid all unnecessary physical and mental suffering and injury.

5.

No experiment should be conducted, where there is an a priori reason to believe that death or disabling injury will occur; except, perhaps, in those experiments where the experimental physicians also serve as subjects.

6.

The degree of risk to be taken should never exceed that determined by the humanitarian importance of the problem to be solved by the experiment.

7.

Proper preparations should be made and adequate facilities provided to protect the experimental subject against even remote possibilities of injury, disability, or death.

8.

The experiment should be conducted only by scientifically qualified persons. The highest degree of skill and care should be required through all stages of the experiment of those who conduct or engage in the experiment.

9.

During the course of the experiment, the human subject should be at liberty to bring the experiment to an end, if he has reached the physical or mental state, where continuation of the experiment seems to him to be impossible.

10.

During the course of the experiment, the scientist in charge must be prepared to terminate the experiment at any stage, if he has probable cause to believe, in the exercise of the good faith, superior skill, and careful judgement required of him, that a continuation of the experiment is likely to result in injury, disability, or death to the experimental subject.

קוד נירנברג
(Hebrew)

1. הסכמה מרצון של הסובייקט האנושי היא חיונית לחלוטין. המשמעות היא שהאדם המעורב צריך להיות בעל כשירות משפטית לתת הסכמה; צריך להיות ממוקם כך שיהיה מסוגל להפעיל סמכות בחירה חופשית, ללא התערבות של כל אלמנט של כוח, הונאה, הונאה, כפיה, הגעת יתר או צורה נסתרת אחרת של אילוץ או כפייה; וצריך להיות בעל ידע והבנה מספקים של מרכיבי הנושא המעורבים כדי לאפשר לו לקבל החלטה מובנת ונאורה. יסוד אחרון זה מחייב כי לפני קבלת החלטה חיובית על ידי הנבדק יש לגלות לו את אופיו, משכו ומטרתו של הניסוי; השיטה והאמצעים שבהם היא אמורה להתנהל; כל אי הנוחות והסיכונים שיש לצפות להם באופן סביר; וההשפעות על בריאותו או האדם שעלולות לנבוע מהשתתפותו בניסוי. החובה והאחריות לברר את טיב ההסכמה מוטלות על כל פרט שיוזם, מנחה או עוסק בניסוי. זוהי חובה ואחריות אישית אשר אין להאציל לאחר ללא עונש.

2. הניסוי צריך להיות כזה שיניב תוצאות פוריות לטובת החברה, בלתי ניתנות לרכישה בשיטות או באמצעי לימוד אחרים, ולא אקראיות ומיותר באופיו.

3. הניסוי צריך להיות מתוכנן ולהתבסס על תוצאות ניסויים בבעלי חיים וידע על ההיסטוריה הטבעית של המחלה או בעיה אחרת הנחקרת, שהתוצאות הצפויות יצדיקו את ביצוע הניסוי.

4. הניסוי צריך להתבצע כך שימנע כל סבל ופציעה פיזית ונפשית מיותרת.

5. אין לערוך ניסוי כאשר יש סיבה אפריורית להאמין שיתרחשו מוות או פציעה משביתה; מלבד, אולי, באותם ניסויים שבהם רופאי הניסוי משמשים גם כנבדקים.

6. מידת הסיכון שיש לקחת לעולם לא תעלה על זו שנקבעת על פי החשיבות ההומ-

ניטרית של הבעיה שתיפתר בניסוי.

7. יש לבצע הכנות מתאימות ולספק מתקנים מתאימים כדי להגן על הנבדק מפני אפשרויות רחוקות אפילו של פציעה, נכות או מוות.

8. הניסוי צריך להתבצע רק על ידי אנשים בעלי הכשרה מדעית. יש לדרוש את המיומנות והזהירות הגבוהה ביותר בכל שלבי הניסוי של אלה שעורכים או עוסקים בניסוי.

9. במהלך הניסוי הנבדק צריך להיות חופשי להביא את הניסוי לסיומו אם הגיע למצב הפיזי או הנפשי שבו המשך הניסוי נראה לו בלתי אפשרי.

10. במהלך הניסוי על המדען האחראי להיות מוכן להפסיק את הניסוי בכל שלב, אם יש לו סיבה סבירה להאמין, בהפעלת תום הלב, המיומנות העליונה ושיקול הדעת הזהיר הנדרשים ממנו כי המשך של הניסוי עלול לגרום לפציעה, נכות או מוות לנבדק הניסוי.

Der Nürnberger Kodex (German)

1. Die freiwillige Zustimmung der Versuchsperson ist unbedingt erforderlich. Das heißt, dass die betreffende Person im juristischen Sinne fähig sein muss, ihre Einwilligung zu geben; dass sie in der Lage sein muss, unbeeinflusst durch Gewalt, Betrug, List, Druck, Vortäuschung oder irgendeine andere Form der Überredung oder des Zwanges, von ihrem Urteilsvermögen Gebrauch zu machen; dass sie das betreffende Gebiet in seinen Einzelheiten hinreichend kennen und verstehen muss, um eine verständige und informierte Entscheidung treffen zu können. Diese letzte Bedingung macht es notwendig, dass der Versuchsperson vor der Einholung ihrer Zustimmung das Wesen, die Länge und der Zweck des Versuches klargemacht werden; sowie die Methode und die Mittel, welche angewendet werden sollen, alle Unannehmlichkeiten und Gefahren, welche mit Fug zu erwarten sind, und die Folgen für ihre Gesundheit oder ihre Person, welche sich aus der Teilnahme ergeben mögen. Die Pflicht und Verantwortlichkeit, den Wert der Zustimmung festzustellen, obliegt jedem, der den Versuch anordnet, leitet oder ihn durchführt. Dies ist eine persönliche Pflicht und Verantwortlichkeit, welche nicht straflos an andere weitergegeben werden kann.

2. Der Versuch muss so gestaltet sein, dass fruchtbare Ergebnisse für das Wohl der Gesellschaft zu erwarten sind, welche nicht durch andere Forschungsmittel oder Methoden zu erlangen sind. Er darf seiner Natur nach nicht willkürlich oder überflüssig sein.

3. Der Versuch ist so zu planen und auf Ergebnissen von Tierversuchen und naturkundlichem Wissen über die Krankheit oder das Forschungsproblem aufzubauen, dass die zu erwartenden Ergebnisse die Durchführung des Versuchs rechtfertigen werden.

4. Der Versuch ist so auszuführen, dass alles unnötige körperliche und seelische Leiden und Schädigungen vermieden werden.

5. Kein Versuch darf durchgeführt werden, wenn von vornherein mit Fug angenommen werden kann, dass es zum Tod oder einem dauernden Schaden führen wird, höchstens jene Versuche ausgenommen, bei welchen der Versuchsleiter gleichzeitig als Versuchsperson dient.

6. Die Gefährdung darf niemals über jene Grenzen hinausgehen, die durch die humanitäre Bedeutung des zu lösenden Problems vorgegeben sind.

7. Es ist für ausreichende Vorbereitung und geeignete Vorrichtungen Sorge zu tragen, um die Versuchsperson auch vor der geringsten Möglichkeit von Verletzung, bleibendem Schaden oder Tod zu schützen.

8. Der Versuch darf nur von wissenschaftlich qualifizierten Personen durchgeführt werden. Größte Geschicklichkeit und Vorsicht sind auf allen Stufen des Versuchs von denjenigen zu verlangen, die den Versuch leiten oder durchführen.

9. Während des Versuches muss der Versuchsperson freigestellt bleiben, den Versuch zu beenden, wenn sie körperlich oder psychisch einen Punkt erreicht hat, an dem ihr seine Fortsetzung unmöglich erscheint.

10. Im Verlauf des Versuchs muss der Versuchsleiter jederzeit darauf vorbereitet sein, den Versuch abzubrechen, wenn er auf Grund des von ihm verlangten guten Glaubens, seiner

besonderen Erfahrung und seines sorgfältigen Urteils vermuten muss, dass eine Fortsetzung des Versuches eine Verletzung, eine bleibende Schädigung oder den Tod der Versuchsperson zur Folge haben könnte.

纽伦堡法典
(Chinese)

1. 人类主体的自愿同意是绝对必要的。这意味着有关人员应具有给予同意的法律能力；应处于能够行使自由选择权的位置，而不受任何武力、欺诈、欺骗、胁迫、过度扩张或其他不可告人的约束或胁迫形式的干预；并且应该对所涉及的主题的元素有足够的知识和理解，以使他能够做出理解和开明的决定。后一个要素要求在实验对象接受肯定的决定之前，应该让他知道实验的性质、持续时间和目的；进行的方法和手段；合理预期的所有不便和危险；以及他参与实验可能对他的健康或人身造成的影响。确定同意质量的义务和责任在于发起、指导或参与实验的每个人。这是一项个人义务和责任，不得将其委托给他人而不受惩罚。

2. 实验应能产生有益于社会的丰硕成果，是其他研究方法或手段无法获得的，不具有随机性和不必要性。

3. 实验的设计应基于动物实验的结果和对疾病自然史或其他研究问题的了解，以使预期结果能够证明实验的执行是合理的。

4. 实验应避免一切不必要的身心痛苦和伤害。

5. 不得进行有先验理由相信会发生死亡或致残伤害的实验；或许，在那些实验医生也作为受试者的实验中。

6. 所承担的风险程度不应超过实验所要解决的问题的人道

主义重要性所决定的程度。

7. 应做好适当的准备并提供足够的设施，以保护实验对象免受伤害、残疾或死亡的微小可能性。

8. 实验只能由具有科学资格的人员进行。进行或参与实验的人在实验的所有阶段都应具备最高程度的技能和谨慎。

9. 在实验过程中，如果人类受试者已经达到他认为不可能继续实验的身体或精神状态，他应该可以自由地结束实验。

10. 在实验过程中，负责科学家必须准备好在任何阶段终止实验，如果他有合理的理由相信，根据他所要求的善意、卓越的技能和谨慎的判断，继续的实验可能导致实验对象受伤、残疾或死亡。

नूर्नबर्ग कोड
(Hindi)

1. मानव विषय की स्वैच्छिक सहमति नितांत आवश्यक है। इसका मतलब है कि इसमें शामिल व्यक्ति के पास सहमति देने की कानूनी क्षमता होनी चाहिए; बल, धोखाधड़ी, छल, दबाव, अतिरेक, या किसी अन्य प्रकार की बाधा या जबरदस्ती के हस्तक्षेप के बिना, अपनी पसंद की स्वतंत्र शक्ति का प्रयोग करने में सक्षम होने के लिए स्थित होना चाहिए; और इसमें शामिल विषय वस्तु के तत्वों का पर्याप्त ज्ञान और समझ होनी चाहिए ताकि वह एक समझ और प्रबुद्ध निर्णय लेने में सक्षम हो सके। इस बाद के तत्व की आवश्यकता है कि प्रयोगात्मक विषय द्वारा सकारात्मक निर्णय की स्वीकृति से पहले उसे प्रयोग की प्रकृति, अवधि और उद्देश्य से अवगत कराया जाना चाहिए; विधि और साधन जिसके द्वारा इसे संचालित किया जाना है; सभी असुविधाओं और खतरों की उचित रूप से अपेक्षा की जानी चाहिए; और उसके स्वास्थ्य या व्यक्ति पर प्रभाव जो संभवतः प्रयोग में उसकी भागीदारी से आ सकता है। सहमति की गुणवत्ता का पता लगाने के लिए कर्तव्य और जिम्मेदारी प्रत्येक व्यक्ति पर होती है जो प्रयोग शुरू करता है, निर्देशित करता है या इसमें संलग्न होता है। यह एक व्यक्तिगत कर्तव्य और जिम्मेदारी है जिसे किसी दूसरे को दण्ड से मुक्ति के साथ नहीं सौंपा जा सकता है।

2. प्रयोग ऐसा होना चाहिए जिससे समाज की भलाई के लिए फलदायी परिणाम मिले, अन्य तरीकों या अध्ययन के माध्यम से अप्राप्य, और प्रकृति में यादृच्छिक और अनावश्यक नहीं।

3. प्रयोग इस तरह से डिजाइन किया जाना चाहिए और पशु प्रयोग के परिणामों और अध्ययन के तहत बीमारी या अन्य समस्या के प्राकृतिक इतिहास के ज्ञान पर आधारित होना चाहिए ताकि प्रत्याशित परिणाम प्रयोग के प्रदर्शन को सही ठहरा सकें।

4. प्रयोग इस प्रकार किया जाना चाहिए कि सभी अनावश्यक शारीरिक और मानसिक पीड़ा और चोट से बचा जा सके।

5. कोई भी प्रयोग नहीं किया जाना चाहिए जहां यह मानने का कोई प्राथमिक कारण हो कि मृत्यु या अक्षम करने वाली चोट लगेगी; सिवाय, शायद, उन प्रयोगों में जहां प्रायोगिक चिकित्सक भी विषयों के रूप में काम करते हैं।

6. प्रयोग द्वारा हल की जाने वाली समस्या के मानवीय महत्व द्वारा निर्धारित जोखिम की डिग्री कभी भी अधिक नहीं होनी चाहिए।

7. उचित तैयारी की जानी चाहिए और प्रायोगिक विषय को चोट, विकलांगता या मृत्यु की दूर-दूर तक की संभावनाओं से बचाने के लिए पर्याप्त सुविधाएं प्रदान की जानी चाहिए।

8. प्रयोग केवल वैज्ञानिक रूप से योग्य व्यक्तियों द्वारा ही किया जाना चाहिए। प्रयोग करने वाले या प्रयोग में संलग्न होने वालों के प्रयोग के सभी चरणों के माध्यम से उच्चतम स्तर के कौशल और देखभाल की आवश्यकता होनी चाहिए।

9. प्रयोग के दौरान मानव विषय को प्रयोग को समाप्त करने के लिए स्वतंत्र होना चाहिए यदि वह शारीरिक या मानसिक स्थिति में पहुंच गया है जहां प्रयोग जारी रखना उसे असंभव लगता है।

10. प्रयोग के दौरान, प्रभारी वैज्ञानिक को किसी भी स्तर पर प्रयोग को समाप्त करने के लिए तैयार रहना चाहिए, यदि उसके पास विश्वास करने का संभावित कारण है, तो उसके लिए आवश्यक सद्भाव, श्रेष्ठ कौशल और सावधानीपूर्वक निर्णय की आवश्यकता है कि एक निरंतरता प्रयोग के परिणामस्वरूप प्रायोगिक विषय को चोट, विकलांगता या मृत्यु होने की संभावना है।

El Código de Nuremberg (Spanish)

1. El consentimiento voluntario del sujeto humano es absolutamente esencial. Esto quiere decir que la persona afectada deberá tener capacidad legal para consentir; deberá estar en situación tal que pueda ejercer plena libertad de elección, sin impedimento alguno de fuerza, fraude, engaño, intimidación, promesa o cualquier otra forma de coacción o amenaza; y deberá tener información y conocimiento suficientes de los elementos del correspondiente experimento, de modo que pueda entender lo que decide. Este último elemento exige que, antes de aceptar una respuesta afirmativa por parte de un sujeto experimental, el investigador tiene que haberle dado a conocer la naturaleza, duración y propósito del experimento; los métodos y medios conforme a los que se llevará a cabo; los inconvenientes y riesgos que razonablemente pueden esperarse; y los efectos que para su salud o personalidad podrían derivarse de su participación en el experimento. El deber y la responsabilidad de evaluar la calidad del consentimiento corren de la cuenta de todos y cada uno de los individuos que inician o dirigen el experimento o que colaboran en él. es un deber y una responsabilidad personal que no puede ser impunemente delegado en otro.

2. El experimento debería ser tal que prometiera dar resultados beneficiosos para el bienestar de la sociedad, y que no pudieran ser obtenidos por otros medios de estudio. No podrán ser de naturaleza caprichosa o innecesaria.

3. El experimento deberá diseñarse y basarse sobre los datos de la experimentación animal previa y sobre el conocimiento de la

historia natural de la enfermedad y de otros problemas en estudio que puedan prometer resultados que justifiquen la realización del experimento.

4. El experimento deberá llevarse a cabo de modo que evite todo sufrimiento o daño físico o mental innecesario.

5. No se podrán realizar experimentos de los que haya razones a priori para creer que puedan producir la muerte o daños incapacitantes graves; excepto, quizás, en aquellos experimentos en los que los mismos experimentadores sirvan como sujetos.

6. El grado de riesgo que se corre nunca podrá exceder el determinado por la importancia humanitaria del problema que el experimento pretende resolver.

7. Deben tomarse las medidas apropiadas y se proporcionaran los dispositivos adecuados para proteger al sujeto de las posibilidades, aun de las más remotas, de lesión, incapacidad o muerte.

8. Los experimentos deberían ser realizados sólo por personas cualificadas científicamente. Deberá exigirse de los que dirigen o participan en el experimento el grado más alto de competencia y solicitud a lo largo de todas sus fases.

9. En el curso del experimento el sujeto será libre de hacer terminar el experimento, si considera que ha llegado a un estado físico o mental en que le parece imposible continuar en él.

10. En el curso del experimento el científico responsable debe estar dispuesto a ponerle fin en cualquier momento, si tiene razones para creer, en el ejercicio de su buena fe, de su habilidad comprobada y de su juicio clínico, que la continuación del experimento puede probablemente dar por resultado la lesión, la incapacidad o la muerte del sujeto experimental.

Le Code de Nuremberg (French)

1. Le consentement volontaire du sujet humain est absolument essentiel. Cela signifie que la personne concernée doit avoir la capacité juridique de donner son consentement ; doit être situé de manière à pouvoir exercer son libre choix, sans l'intervention d'aucun élément de force, de fraude, de tromperie, de contrainte, d'excès ou de toute autre forme ultérieure de contrainte ou de coercition ; et doit avoir une connaissance et une compréhension suffisantes des éléments du sujet concerné pour lui permettre de prendre une décision éclairée et éclairée. Ce dernier élément exige qu'avant l'acceptation d'une décision affirmative par le sujet expérimental, on lui fasse connaître la nature, la durée et le but de l'expérience ; la méthode et les moyens par lesquels elle doit être menée ; tous les inconvénients et dangers auxquels on peut raisonnablement s'attendre ; et les effets sur sa santé ou sur sa personne qui pourraient résulter de sa participation à l'expérience. Le devoir et la responsabilité de s'assurer de la qualité du consentement incombent à chaque individu qui initie, dirige ou s'engage dans l'expérience. C'est un devoir et une responsabilité personnels qui ne peuvent être impunément délégués à un autre.

2. L'expérience doit être telle qu'elle donne des résultats fructueux pour le bien de la société, impossibles à obtenir par d'autres méthodes ou moyens d'étude, et non aléatoires et inutiles par nature.

3. L'expérience doit être conçue et basée sur les résultats de l'expérimentation animale et sur une connaissance de l'histoire naturelle de la maladie ou d'un autre problème à l'étude, de sorte que les résultats escomptés justifient la réalisation de l'expérience.

4. L'expérience doit être menée de manière à éviter toutes souffrances et blessures physiques et mentales inutiles.

5. Aucune expérience ne doit être menée lorsqu'il existe une raison a priori de croire qu'un décès ou une blessure invalidante surviendra; sauf, peut-être, dans les expériences où les médecins expérimentateurs servent aussi de sujets.

6. Le degré de risque à prendre ne doit jamais dépasser celui déterminé par l'importance humanitaire du problème à résoudre par l'expérience.

7. Des préparatifs appropriés doivent être faits et des installations adéquates doivent être fournies pour protéger le sujet expérimental contre les possibilités, même lointaines, de blessure, d'invalidité ou de décès.

8. L'expérience ne doit être menée que par des personnes scientifiquement qualifiées. Le plus haut degré de compétence et de soin devrait être requis à toutes les étapes de l'expérience de ceux qui mènent ou s'engagent dans l'expérience.

9. Au cours de l'expérience, le sujet humain doit être libre de mettre fin à l'expérience s'il a atteint l'état physique ou mental où la poursuite de l'expérience lui paraît impossible.

10. Au cours de l'expérience, le scientifique responsable doit être prêt à mettre fin à l'expérience à n'importe quel stade, s'il a des raisons probables de croire, dans l'exercice de la bonne foi, une habileté supérieure et un jugement prudent requis de lui qu'une poursuite de l'expérience est susceptible d'entraîner des blessures, une invalidité ou la mort du sujet expérimental.

قانون نورمبرغ
(Arabic)

1. الموافقة الطوعية للفرد البشري ضرورية للغاية. وهذا يعني أن الشخص المعني يجب أن يتمتع بالأهلية القانونية لمنح الموافقة ؛ يجب أن يكون في وضع يسمح له بممارسة حرية الاختيار ، دون تدخل أي عنصر من عناصر القوة ، أو الاحتيال ، أو الخداع ، أو الإكراه ، أو التجاوز ، أو أي شكل خفي من أشكال القهر أو الإكراه ؛ ويجب أن يكون لديه معرفة وفهم كافيين لعناصر الموضوع المعني لتمكينه من اتخاذ قرار مستنير وتفهم. يتطلب هذا العنصر الأخير أنه قبل قبول قرار إيجابي من قبل الموضوع التجريبي ، يجب أن يكون معروفًا له طبيعة التجربة ومدتها والغرض منها ؛ الطريقة والوسائل التي سيتم من خلالها إجراؤها ؛ جميع المضايقات والمخاطر التي يمكن توقعها بشكل معقول ؛ والآثار التي قد تنجم عن مشاركته في التجربة على صحته أو شخصه. يقع واجب ومسؤولية التحقق من جودة الموافقة على عاتق كل فرد يبدأ التجربة أو يوجهها أو يشارك فيها. إنه واجب شخصي ومسؤولية لا يجوز تفويضها إلى شخص آخر دون عقاب.

2. أن تكون التجربة من النوع الذي يعطي نتائج مثمرة لصالح المجتمع ، لا يمكن تحقيقه بوسائل أو طرق أخرى للدراسة ، وليست عشوائية وغير ضرورية بطبيعتها.

3. يجب أن تكون التجربة مصممة بحيث تستند إلى نتائج التجارب على الحيوانات ومعرفة التاريخ الطبيعي للمرض أو أي مشكلة أخرى قيد الدراسة بحيث تكون النتائج المتوقعة تبرر أداء التجربة.

4. يجب إجراء التجربة بحيث يتم تجنب كل المعاناة الجسدية والعقلية والإصابات غير الضرورية.

5. لا ينبغي إجراء أي تجربة إذا كان هناك سبب مسبق للاعتقاد بحدوث وفاة أو إصابة معيقة. ربما باستثناء تلك التجارب حيث يعمل الأطباء التجريبيون أيضًا كمواضيع.

6. يجب ألا تتجاوز درجة المخاطرة التي يجب اتخاذها الدرجة التي تحددها الأهمية الإنسانية للمشكلة التي سيتم حلها من خلال التجربة.

7. يجب إجراء الاستعدادات المناسبة وتوفير التسهيلات الكافية لحماية موضوع التجربة حتى من الاحتمالات البعيدة للإصابة أو العجز أو الوفاة.

8. أن تجرى التجربة فقط من قبل أشخاص مؤهلين علمياً. يجب أن تكون أعلى درجة من المهارة والعناية مطلوبة خلال جميع مراحل التجربة لأولئك الذين أجروا التجربة أو شاركوا فيها.

9. خلال فترة التجربة ، يجب أن يكون الإنسان حراً في إنهاء التجربة إذا كان قد وصل إلى الحالة الجسدية أو العقلية حيث يبدو له أن استمرار التجربة مستحيل.

10. أثناء التجربة ، يجب أن يكون العالم المسؤول مستعدًا لإنهاء التجربة في أي مرحلة ، إذا كان لديه سبب محتمل للاعتقاد ، في ممارسة حسن النية والمهارة الفائقة والحكم الدقيق المطلوب منه استمرار من المحتمل أن تؤدي التجربة إلى إصابة أو عجز أو وفاة لموضوع التجربة.

Нюрнбергский кодекс (Russian)

1. Абсолютно необходимым условием проведения эксперимента на человеке является добровольное согласие последнего. Это означает, что лицо, вовлекаемое в эксперимент в качестве испытуемого, должно иметь законное право давать такое согласие; иметь возможность осуществлять свободный выбор и не испытывать на себе влияние каких-либо элементов насилия, обмана, мошенничества, хитрости или других скрытых форм давления или принуждения; обладать знаниями, достаточными для того, чтобы понять суть эксперимента и принять осознанное решение. Последнее требует, чтобы до принятия утвердительного решения о возможности своего участия в том или ином эксперименте испытуемый был информирован о характере, продолжительности и цели данного эксперимента; о методах и способах его проведения; обо всех предполагаемых неудобствах и опасностях, связанных с проведением эксперимента, и, наконец, возможных последствиях для физического или психического здоровья испытуемого, могущих возникнуть в результате его участия в эксперименте. Обязанность и ответственность за выяснение качества полученного согласия лежит на каждом, кто инициирует, руководит или занимается проведением данного эксперимента. Это персональная обязанность и ответственность каждого такого лица, которая не может быть безнаказанно переложена на другое лицо.

2. Эксперимент должен приносить обществу положительные результаты, недостижимые другими методами или способами исследования; он не должен носить случайный, необязательный по своей сути характер.

3. Эксперимент должен основываться на данных, полученных в лабораторных исследованиях на животных,

знании истории развития данного заболевания или других изучаемых проблем. Его проведение должно быть так организовано, чтобы ожидаемые результаты оправдывали сам факт его проведения.

4. При проведении эксперимента необходимо избегать всех излишних физических и психических страданий и повреждений.

5. Ни один эксперимент не должен проводиться в случае, если "a priori" есть основания предполагать возможность смерти или инвалидизирующего ранения испытуемого; исключением, возможно, могут являться случаи, когда врачи исследователи выступают в качестве испытуемых при проведении своих экспериментов.

6. Степень риска, связанного с проведением эксперимента, никогда не должна превышать гуманитарной важности проблемы, на решение которой направлен данный эксперимент.

7. Эксперименту должна предшествовать соответствующая подготовка, и его проведение должно быть обеспечено оборудованием, необходимым для защиты испытуемого от малейшей возможности ранения, инвалидности или смерти.

8. Эксперимент должен проводиться только лицами, имеющими научную квалификацию. На всех стадиях эксперимента от тех, кто проводит его или занят в нем, требуется максимум внимания и профессионализма.

9. В ходе проведения эксперимента испытуемый должен иметь возможность остановить его, если, по его мнению, его физическое или психическое состояние делает невозможным продолжение эксперимента.

10. В ходе эксперимента исследователь, отвечающий за его проведение, должен быть готов прекратить его на любой стадии, если профессиональные соображения, добросовестность и осторожность в суждениях, требуемые от него, дают основания полагать, что продолжение эксперимента может привести к ранению, инвалидности или смерти испытуемого.

O Código de Nuremberg
(Portuguese)

1. O consentimento voluntário do sujeito humano é absolutamente essencial. Isso significa que a pessoa envolvida deve ter capacidade legal para dar consentimento; deve estar situado de modo a poder exercer o livre poder de escolha, sem a intervenção de qualquer elemento de força, fraude, engano, coação, exagero ou outra forma ulterior de coação ou coação; e deve ter conhecimento e compreensão suficientes dos elementos do assunto em questão, de modo a capacitá-lo a tomar uma decisão compreensiva e esclarecida. Este último elemento requer que, antes da aceitação de uma decisão afirmativa pelo sujeito do experimento, lhe seja dado conhecimento da natureza, duração e propósito do experimento; o método e os meios pelos quais ela deve ser conduzida; todos os inconvenientes e perigos razoavelmente esperados; e os efeitos sobre sua saúde ou pessoa que podem vir de sua participação no experimento. O dever e a responsabilidade de verificar a qualidade do consentimento recai sobre cada indivíduo que inicia, dirige ou se envolve no experimento. É um dever e uma responsabilidade pessoal que não pode ser delegada a outrem impunemente.

2. A experiência deve ser tal que produza resultados frutíferos para o bem da sociedade, inalcançáveis por outros métodos ou meios de estudo, e não de natureza aleatória e desnecessária.

3. A experiência deve ser concebida de tal forma e baseada nos resultados da experimentação animal e no conhecimento da história natural da doença ou outro problema em estudo que os resultados previstos justifiquem a realização da experiência.

4. O experimento deve ser conduzido de modo a evitar todo sofrimento e lesões físicas e mentais desnecessárias.

5. Nenhum experimento deve ser conduzido onde houver uma razão a priori para acreditar que a morte ou lesão incapacitante ocorrerá; exceto, talvez, naqueles experimentos em que os médicos experimentais também servem como sujeitos.

6. O grau de risco a ser assumido nunca deve exceder aquele determinado pela importância humanitária do problema a ser resolvido pelo experimento.

7. Os preparativos apropriados devem ser feitos e as instalações adequadas devem ser fornecidas para proteger o sujeito experimental mesmo contra possibilidades remotas de lesão, incapacidade ou morte.

8. O experimento deve ser conduzido apenas por pessoas cientificamente qualificadas. O mais alto grau de habilidade e cuidado deve ser exigido em todos os estágios do experimento daqueles que conduzem ou se envolvem no experimento.

9. Durante o curso do experimento, o sujeito humano deve ter a liberdade de terminar o experimento se ele atingiu o estado físico ou mental em que a continuação do experimento lhe parece impossível.

10. Durante o curso do experimento, o cientista responsável deve estar preparado para encerrar o experimento em qualquer estágio, se ele tiver motivos prováveis para acreditar, no exercício da boa fé, habilidade superior e julgamento cuidadoso exigido dele que uma continuação do experimento é susceptível de resultar em lesão, incapacidade ou morte para o sujeito experimental.

Il Codice di Norimberga (Italian)

1. Il consenso volontario del soggetto umano è assolutamente indispensabile. Ciò significa che la persona coinvolta dovrebbe avere la capacità giuridica di dare il consenso; dovrebbe essere situato in modo da poter esercitare il libero potere di scelta, senza l'intervento di alcun elemento di forza, frode, inganno, costrizione, smisurato, o altra ulteriore forma di costrizione o coercizione; e dovrebbe avere sufficiente conoscenza e comprensione degli elementi dell'argomento in questione da consentirgli di prendere una decisione comprensiva e illuminata. Quest'ultimo elemento richiede che prima dell'accettazione di una decisione affermativa da parte del soggetto sperimentale gli venga comunicata la natura, la durata e lo scopo dell'esperimento; il metodo e i mezzi con cui deve essere condotto; tutti gli inconvenienti e pericoli ragionevolmente prevedibili; e gli effetti sulla sua salute o persona che potrebbero derivare dalla sua partecipazione all'esperimento. Il dovere e la responsabilità di accertare la qualità del consenso spetta a ciascun individuo che avvia, dirige o partecipa all'esperimento. È un dovere e una responsabilità personali che non possono essere delegati ad altri impunemente.

2. L'esperimento deve essere tale da produrre risultati fruttuosi per il bene della società, non ottenibili con altri metodi o mezzi di studio, e di natura non casuale e non necessaria.

3. L'esperimento dovrebbe essere progettato e basato sui risultati della sperimentazione animale e sulla conoscenza della storia naturale della malattia o di altri problemi oggetto di studio che i

risultati previsti giustifichino l'esecuzione dell'esperimento.

4. L'esperimento dovrebbe essere condotto in modo da evitare tutte le sofferenze e le lesioni fisiche e mentali non necessarie.

5. Nessun esperimento dovrebbe essere condotto laddove vi sia un motivo a priori per ritenere che si verificherà la morte o una lesione invalidante; tranne, forse, in quegli esperimenti in cui i medici sperimentali servono anche come soggetti.

6. Il grado di rischio da correre non deve mai superare quello determinato dall'importanza umanitaria del problema da risolvere con l'esperimento.

7. Dovrebbero essere fatti i preparativi adeguati e dovrebbero essere fornite strutture adeguate per proteggere il soggetto sperimentale da possibilità anche remote di lesioni, disabilità o morte.

8. L'esperimento dovrebbe essere condotto solo da persone scientificamente qualificate. Il più alto grado di abilità e cura dovrebbe essere richiesto in tutte le fasi dell'esperimento di coloro che conducono o si impegnano nell'esperimento.

9. Nel corso dell'esperimento il soggetto umano dovrebbe essere libero di portare a termine l'esperimento se ha raggiunto lo stato fisico o mentale in cui la continuazione dell'esperimento gli sembra impossibile.

10. Nel corso dell'esperimento, lo scienziato incaricato deve essere preparato a terminare l'esperimento in qualsiasi momento, se ha motivo di ritenere probabile, nell'esercizio della buona fede, una superiore abilità e un attento giudizio gli richiedessero che una continuazione dell'esperimento rischia di provocare lesioni, invalidità o morte per il soggetto sperimentale.

ニュルンベルク綱領
(Japanese)

1. 被験者の自発的な同意は絶対に不可欠です。これは、関係者が同意を与える法的能力を持っている必要があることを意味します。力、詐欺、欺瞞、脅迫、行き過ぎ、またはその他の潜在的な拘束または強制の要素の介入なしに、自由な選択権を行使できるように位置付けられる必要があります。また、関係する主題の要素について十分な知識と理解を持ち、理解と賢明な決定を下すことができるようにする必要があります。この後者の要素は、実験対象者が肯定的な決定を受け入れる前に、実験の性質、期間、および目的を彼に知らせる必要があることを要求します。それが実施される方法と手段。合理的に予想されるすべての不便と危険。実験への参加から生じる可能性のある彼の健康または人体への影響。同意の質を確認する義務と責任は、実験を開始、指示、または従事する各個人にかかっています。これは個人の義務と責任であり、責任を問われることなく他人に委任することはできません。

2. 実験は、社会の利益のために実りある結果をもたらし、他の方法や研究手段では手に入れることができず、無作為で不必要なものであってはなりません。

3. 実験は、予想される結果が実験の実施を正当化するように、動物実験の結果および研究中の疾患またはその他の問題の自然史に関する知識に基づいて計画されるべきである。

4. 実験は、すべての不必要な身体的および精神的苦痛および損傷を避けるように実施する必要があります。

5. 死亡または障害を引き起こす傷害が発生すると信じる先験的な理由がある場合、実験は実施されるべきではありません。おそらく、実験医師が被験者としても働く実験を除いて。

6. とるべきリスクの程度は、実験によって解決される問題の人道的重要性によって決定されるレベルを超えてはなりません。

7. 怪我、障害、または死亡のわずかな可能性から実験対象者を保護するために、適切な準備を行い、適切な設備を提供する必要があります。

8. 実験は、科学的に資格のある人によってのみ行われるべきです。実験を実施または実施する者は、実験のすべての段階を通じて、最高度の技術と注意を払う必要があります。

9. 実験の過程で、被験者は、実験の継続が不可能と思われる身体的または精神的状態に達した場合、自由に実験を終了できる必要があります。

10. 実験の進行中、担当の科学者は、実験を継続するために必要な誠実さ、優れた技術、および慎重な判断の行使において、信じるに足る理由がある場合、いつでも実験を終了する準備ができていなければなりません。実験の結果、実験対象者に傷害、障害、または死亡が生じる可能性があります。

Additional Reading

Evans, Suzanne - **Hitler's Forgotten Victims: The Holocaust and the Disabled**

Freyhofer, Horst H. - **The Nuremberg Medical Trial: The Holocaust and the Origin of the Nuremberg Medical Code**

Goldensohn, Leon - **The Nuremberg Interviews**

Grodin, Michael A. - **The Nazi Doctors and the Nuremberg Code: Human Rights in Human Experimentation**

Kennedy Jr, Robert F. - **The Real Anthony Fauci**

Kennedy Jr, Robert F. - **A Letter to Liberals: Censorship and COVID: An Attack on Science and American Ideals**

Lifton, Robert J. - **The Nazi Doctors: Medical Killing and the Psychology of Genocide**

McCarthy, Ken - **Unraveling The CoVid Con (2020-2022)**

McCarthy, Ken - **The Nuremberg Code and Its Modern Enemies**

Mitscherlich, Alexander; Mielke, Fred - **Doctors of Infamy**

Proctor, Robert N. - **Racial Hygiene**

Robertson, Michael; Ley, Astrid; Light, Edwina - **The First into the Dark: The Nazi Persecution of the Disabled**

Taylor, Telford - **The Anatomy of the Nuremberg Trials: A Personal Memoir**

Weindling, P. - **Nazi Medicine and the Nuremberg Trials: From Medical Warcrimes to Informed Consent**

An organization dedicated to the issue of medical justice:

Alliance for Human Research Protection
Advancing Voluntary, Informed Consent to Medical Intervention

Visit: ahrp.org

Next Steps...

Help us put this book in the hands of more people

Visit: Nuremberg75.com

Or scan with your phone below:

Additional Titles From Brasscheck Press
Available at Brasscheck.com/books

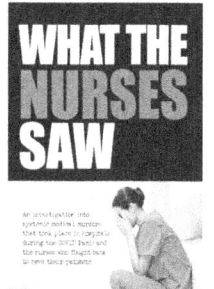

What The Nurses Saw:
An Investigation Into Systemic Medical Murders That Took Place in Hospitals During the COVID Panic and the Nurses Who Fought Back to Save Their Patients

Over 1,000,000 Americans are said to have "died of COVID" between 2020 and 2023. 92% of these deaths occurred in hospitals or other health care facilities. The U.S. despite having approximately 4.2% of the total world population had more reported COVID deaths in absolute terms than any other country and by far measure. This book addresses the so-far unasked question "Why?"

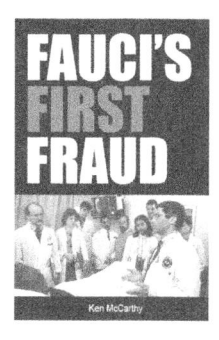

Fauci's First Fraud: The Foundation of Medical Totalitarianism in America

Forty years before the global COVID Panic, U.S. federal bureaucracies like the CDC and NIAID were having trouble justifying their budgets because of the dramatic decline of deaths from infectious diseases.

The solution: The creation of a propaganda machine that successfully floods the news media with hysteria-tinged reports of biological doom while simultaneously shouting down all rational scientific and medical discussion of health issues.

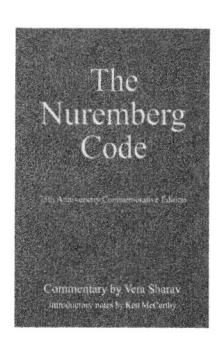

The Nuremberg Code:
75th Anniversary Commemorative Edition

A concise and essential document on the subject of patient rights, drafted in response to many heinous abuses by doctors, nurses, and public health officials during the Nazi regime.
This 75th Anniversary Commemorative Edition of the Nuremberg Code features a moving introduction by Holocaust survivor Vera Sharav and translations of the original Code in 11 languages. The full text of the book is available in German, Russian, Spanish, and French editions, with hopefully more languages to come.

Coming in 2025 — The Nuremberg Code and its Modern Enemies

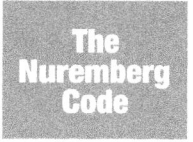

Where did respect for the Nuremberg Code go?

In the middle of the COVID Panic, the 75th anniversary of the Nuremberg Code (2022) came and went without recognition or even mention from anyone in the medical ethics profession.

Meanwhile, a cottage industry of "reporters" sprung up producing a stream of articles about how the Code was out of date, not legally binding, and does not apply to COVID vaccines. This book answers the question "Why?"

Brasscheck.com
In-depth common-sense online reporting since 1997

Made in United States
North Haven, CT
18 February 2025